HORMONAL WEIGHT GAIN (HUNGER PANGS)

"Healthy Eating Habits"

BY

Venita Yvonne Vance

Broad Book Basics

Table of Contents

INTRODUCTION

The distinction between simple weight increase and hormone weight gain is significant. Most of the time, a person can identify the reason(s) for their additional weight gain; often, eating too many unhealthy foods and living a sedentary life are to blame. Hormone weight gain is distinct from other types of weight gain in that the individual is often just as active and hasn't made any dietary changes, yet they are still gaining weight. The quantity of hormone-induced weight gain can occasionally be shocking.

How a person responds to hormonal weight gain can be greatly influenced by attitude. The worst thing a person can do is to accept the weight gain and give in to their hormones.

It's not always simple for someone to maintain their positive attitude, particularly when they are struggling with an unexpected weight increase. Depression and exhaustion are two other prevalent adverse effects of hormonal imbalance, and, to be very honest, they are most likely also brought on by an increase in body mass. The person needs to make an effort to surround oneself with positive, entertaining and motivating people to cope.

When a person is battling with hormone weight gain, diet and exercise are crucial. Eating a healthy, well-balanced diet doesn't harm even if regular diets aren't usually efficient for preventing weight gain brought on by hormones. Working together frequently achieves two goals. The primary benefit of exercise is that it maintains the person's muscles toned and joints flexibility. The second benefit of exercising is that it gets one out of the home, which aids in overcoming depression. Endorphins are released during exercise, and they help speed metabolic metabolism. A high metabolism will aid in the body burning more calories, preventing weight gain, which is unquestionably the intended outcome.

To our dismay, it appears that for the majority of women, the stomach, hips, and waistline tend to be the most preferred regions for additional body fat to be deposited.

Reducing your calorie consumption won't make much of a difference in keeping your yesterday's hourglass figure because calories consumed aren't the perpetrators either.

Popular diets that advocate for calorie intakes of fewer than 1,200 per day might worsen the issue and be harmful to your health!

Instead, hormonal weight gain is a direct result of changes and swings in a woman's hormone levels, and the thickening effect that follows. In other words, your hormones are to thank for that extra belly fat.

There is no doubt that there is a very close connection between hormones and weight growth, and there are four important hormones involved, each of which plays a different function in how and where your body stores body fat.

The first two key things that might affect the status of your hormones are diet and exercise.

Three other significant aspects that affect the status of your hormones and your ability to maintain a healthy body weight are stress, sleep, and nutritional supplements.

It might also be useful to know what NOT to do.

For instance, it's crucial to limit or stay away from excessive amounts of caffeine, alcohol, and other stimulants.

The good news for women is that many of these variables may be adjusted or modified to help them attain the ideal hormonal balance and prevent weight gain due to hormones.

HORMONES THAT CAN CAUSE WEIGHT GAIN

Hormones play a crucial role in your body as chemical messengers.

They support almost all physiological functions, such as metabolism, hunger, and fullness. Some hormones can significantly affect body weight due to their connection to hunger.

Here are some hormones that may have an impact on your weight and advice on how to maintain appropriate levels of each.

Insulin

Your pancreas produces insulin, which is the main hormone used for storage in your body. Insulin encourages the storage of glucose, a simple sugar obtained from meals, in the muscle, liver, and fat cells for later use in healthy humans.

Insulin is secreted by your body in little amounts throughout the day and greater quantities following meals. Depending on your body's present demands, this hormone then transports glucose from meals into your cells for either energy or storage.

Your cells cease reacting to insulin when you have insulin resistance, which is a pretty common disorder. Due to the insulin's inability to transport glucose into your cells, this disorder causes high blood sugar.

To increase glucose absorption, your pancreas subsequently generates more insulin.

Obesity has been related to insulin resistance, and obesity can contribute to other diseases including type 2 diabetes and heart disease.

One might consider insulin sensitivity to be the polar opposite of insulin resistance. It indicates that your cells are insulin-sensitive. So it makes sense to concentrate on lifestyle practices that raise insulin sensitivity, such as the ones listed below.

Tips to improve insulin sensitivity

- Regular exercise, Exercise has been shown to increase insulin sensitivity and reduce insulin resistance when performed at high and moderate intensities.

- Adapt your sleeping patterns. Obesity and insulin resistance are connected to inadequate sleep, whether it is quantity or quality.

- Get additional omega-3 fatty acids. According to research, omega-3 supplements may help persons with metabolic disorders like diabetes have better insulin sensitivity. If supplements aren't your thing, try consuming more fish, nuts, seeds, and plant oils.

- Modify your diet. The Mediterranean diet, which is high in extra-virgin olive oil and healthful fats from nuts and seeds, may help lower insulin resistance. Reducing your consumption of saturated and trans fats may also be beneficial.

- Sustain a healthy weight. Healthy weight loss and weight control may increase insulin sensitivity in overweight individuals.

- Pay attention to low glycemic carbs. Make the majority of your carbs low glycemic and high in fiber rather than trying to completely cut them out of your diet. Whole grains, fruits, vegetables, and legumes are among the examples.

Leptin

Leptin is a hormone that promotes feeling full by signaling your hypothalamus, which controls your appetite, that you are full.

Leptin resistance, however, may occur in obese persons. As a result, your brain doesn't get the signal to quit eating, which eventually leads to overeating.

Your body may then continue to generate leptin until your levels rise.

Leptin resistance may be caused directly by inflammation, gene mutations, or increased leptin synthesis, which can happen with obesity, although the exact reason is unknown.

Tips to improve leptin levels

- Leptin resistance has no known cure, however, several lifestyle modifications might help reduce leptin levels.
- Keep a healthy weight. It's crucial to keep a healthy weight since leptin resistance is linked to obesity. Additionally, evidence points to a possible link between lower body fat and lower leptin levels.
- The caliber of your sleep. In obese patients, leptin levels may be correlated with sleep quality. There are a lot of other reasons to obtain better sleep, even though this link might not be present in those who are not obese.
- Regular exercise. Leptin levels are believed to fall as a result of frequent, consistent exercise.

Overeating may occur in obese persons due to resistance to the hormone leptin, which makes you feel full. According to research, a healthy body weight, frequent exercise, and sound sleep all contribute to reduced leptin levels.

Ghrelin

Leptin and ghrelin are fundamentally opposing hormones. Your hypothalamus receives a signal from the hunger hormone telling it that your stomach is empty and that you need to eat. Its primary purpose is to stimulate hunger.

Ghrelin levels are often greatest before meals and lowest thereafter.

Curiously, studies show that obese individuals have lower ghrelin levels yet are more susceptible to its effects. This sensitivity might result in overeating.

Tips to manage ghrelin levels

- The fact that cutting calories frequently causes your ghrelin levels to rise and leave you feeling hungry is one reason why losing weight can be challenging. Additionally, leptin levels drop and metabolism tends to slow down.
- As a result, the following advice for reducing ghrelin to aid in appetite suppression:
- Preserve a healthy body weight. Your sensitivity to ghrelin may grow as a result of obesity, which would therefore increase your hunger.
- Make an effort to obtain great rest. Increases in ghrelin, overeating and weight gain can result from a lack of sleep.
- Eat consistently. Ghrelin levels are at their peak just before a meal, so pay attention to your hunger cues and eat when it comes.

The effects of the hunger hormone ghrelin may be felt more keenly by obese people. According to research, controlling this hormone is aided by keeping a moderate body weight and giving sleep priority.

Cortisol

Your adrenal glands create cortisol, sometimes known as the stress hormone.

This hormone causes an increase in energy and heart rate while under stress. The phrase "fight or flight" refers to the production of the hormones cortisol and adrenaline.

Although your body needs to release cortisol under harmful circumstances, prolonged high amounts can cause several health problems, including diabetes, heart disease, poor energy, high blood pressure, sleep disorders, and weight gain.

High cortisol levels may be caused by several lifestyle choices, such as insufficient sleep, ongoing stress, and eating a lot of high-glycemic meals.

Additionally, a negative feedback loop is created by the fact that obesity not only raises cortisol levels but that high levels may also lead to weight increase.

Tips for lowering cortisol levels

Here are some lifestyle changes that may help manage cortisol levels:

- Improve sleep. High cortisol levels may be caused by long-term sleep problems such as insomnia, sleep apnea, and irregular sleeping patterns (like those of shift workers). Concentrate on creating a consistent bedtime and sleep regimen.

- Regular exercise High-intensity exercise briefly raises cortisol levels, while regular exercise typically lowers them by enhancing general health and reducing stress.

- Engage in mindfulness. There has to be more research, however, it appears that mindfulness practice frequently decreases cortisol levels. Make meditation a regular part of your regimen.

- Preserve a healthy body weight. Maintaining a reasonable weight may assist keep levels in line because obesity has been linked to an increase in cortisol levels, and high cortisol levels have been linked to weight growth.

- Eat a balanced diet. Research has shown that diets high in added sugars, refined grains, and saturated fat may lead to higher cortisol levels. Additionally, following the Mediterranean diet may help lower cortisol levels.

Although cortisol is a vital hormone, persistently excessive amounts can cause diseases including diabetes, heart disease, and obesity. Your levels may be lowered by maintaining a nutritious diet, exercising frequently, getting enough sleep, and engaging in mindfulness exercises.

Estrogen

Estrogen is a sex hormone that controls the immunological, skeletal, and circulatory systems in addition to the female reproductive system.

The levels of this hormone fluctuate throughout the menstrual cycle and during many life phases, including pregnancy, lactation, and menopause.

High estrogen levels, which are frequently found in obese individuals, are linked to an increased risk of some malignancies and other chronic disorders.

Conversely, low levels, which are often associated with aging, perimenopause, and menopause, may have an impact on body weight and body fat, raising your chance of developing chronic illnesses.

Low estrogen levels frequently result in central obesity, which is a buildup of weight around the body's trunk. Other health issues including excessive blood sugar, high blood pressure, and heart disease may result from this.

By making lifestyle adjustments, especially by keeping a healthy body weight, you can reduce your chance of developing many of these health issues.

Tips to maintain healthy estrogen levels

To keep estrogen levels at a healthy equilibrium, try some of these techniques:

- Attempt to control your weight. Due to low estrogen levels in women between the ages of 55 and 75, weight loss or maintenance may lower the risk of heart disease. Research also supports maintaining a healthy weight to prevent chronic illnesses in general.
- Regular exercise. You can feel less capable of exercising if you have low estrogen levels. Nevertheless, regular exercise is still essential to help with weight control during times of low estrogen secretion, such as menopause.

- Maintain a healthy diet. It has been demonstrated that diets heavy in red meat, processed foods, sweets, and refined grains enhance estrogen levels, which may increase your chance of developing chronic diseases. As a result, you might want to restrict how often you eat certain items.

Maintaining a healthy lifestyle can help to reduce your risk of the disease since estrogen levels, which are affected by both high and low sex activity, can cause weight gain.

Neuropeptide Y

In reaction to fasting or stress, your brain and nervous system create the hormone neuropeptide Y (NPY), which increases hunger and lowers energy expenditure.

NPY is linked to obesity and weight gain because it may boost food consumption.

It is activated in fat tissue, where it may increase fat storage, cause abdominal obesity, and result in metabolic syndrome, which raises the chance of developing chronic illnesses.

According to research, NPY's processes that produce obesity may also trigger an inflammatory response, making existing medical issues worse.

Tips for maintaining low NPY levels

Here are some tips for maintaining healthy levels of NPY:

- Exercise. There is conflicting evidence, although some studies point to the possibility that regular exercise may help lower NPY levels.
- Consume a healthy diet. Although additional study is required, high fat, high sugar diets may raise NPY levels; therefore, you may want to think about reducing your intake of these foods.

NPY is a hormone that increases hunger and has been linked to obesity. Regular exercise and a good diet could be beneficial for maintaining healthy levels.

Glucagon-like peptide-1

A hormone called Glucagon-like peptide-1 (GLP-1) is created in the gut when food enters the intestines. It is crucial for stabilizing blood sugar levels and promoting satiety.

According to research, GLP-1 signaling may be compromised in obese persons.

As a result, GLP-1 is included in drugs, especially those prescribed for persons with diabetes, to help patients lose weight and shrink their waistlines.

Tips for keeping GLP-1 levels in check

Here are some tips to help maintain healthy levels of GLP-1:

- Eat a lot of protein. Yogurt and other high-protein foods, such as whey protein, have been demonstrated to raise GLP-1 levels.
- Think about consuming probiotics. Probiotics may raise GLP-1 levels, according to a preliminary study, but further human studies are required. It's

also important to see a healthcare provider before beginning any new supplements.

GLP-1 is a hormone that causes fullness, although obese people may not be as susceptible to its effects. Try to eat a well-rounded diet with lots of protein to keep your GLP-1 levels in check.

Cholecystokinin

Cholecystokinin (CCK), like GLP-1, is a hormone that your gut produces after a meal to make you feel full. It is necessary for digestion, the synthesis of proteins, the creation of energy, and other biological processes. Leptin, a hormone that signals fullness, is also released more often.

People who are obese may be less sensitive to the effects of CCK, which might result in persistent overeating. A negative feedback loop might be created as a result, further decreasing CCK sensitivity.

Tips for increasing CCK levels

Here are some tips for maintaining healthy levels of CCK:

- Consume a lot of protein. According to certain studies, a high-protein diet may help raise CCK levels and, as a result, fullness.
- Exercise. Despite the paucity of study, some data point to the benefits of regular exercise for raising CCK levels.

People with obesity may develop sensitivity to the fullness hormone CCK. This could result in overeating. For a diet high in protein and frequent exercise to keep CCK levels in check.

Peptide YY

Another gut hormone that suppresses appetite is peptide YY (PYY).

PYY levels may be reduced in obese individuals, which may cause an increase in hunger and overeating. It is thought that adequate levels significantly contribute to lowering food intake and lowering the risk of obesity.

Tips for raising PYY levels

Here are some ways to keep PYY at a healthy level in your body:

- Maintain a balanced diet. Protein consumption in large amounts may support normal PYY levels and satiety. Furthermore, the paleo diet, which is high in fruits, vegetables, and protein, may increase PYY levels, although further study is required.
- Exercise. Even though there is contrary evidence about exercise and PYY levels, being active is usually good for your health.

Low levels of PYY, a hormone that signals fullness, may be present in obese people. A high-protein diet and regular exercise may help increase levels.

The levels of these hormones may be optimized by specific lifestyle practices, according to research, but it's crucial to check with a healthcare provider if you think your hormones may be out of balance.

Overall, maintaining a balanced diet, placing a high priority on sleep, and engaging in regular exercise may improve your general health and lower your chance of developing chronic diseases.

WHAT IS THE MEANING OF HORMONAL IMBALANCE

What Are Hormones?

Hormones are substances that communicate with your organs, skin, muscles, and other tissues through your blood to coordinate various bodily activities. These messages instruct your body on what to do and when. Hormones are necessary for both life and wellness.

In the human body, there are currently approximately 50 hormones known to science.

Your endocrine system is made up of the majority of tissues (mostly glands) that produce and release hormones. Numerous bodily functions are controlled by hormones, including:

- Metabolism.
- Homeostasis (constant internal balance).
- Growth and development.
- Sexual function.
- Reproduction.
- Sleep-wake cycle.
- Mood.

What Is A Hormonal Imbalance?

When one or more of your hormones are either produced in excess or lacking in quality, you have a hormonal imbalance. It's a general phrase that can refer to a wide range of hormonal disorders.

Hormones are potent messengers. For several hormones, even a minor excess or deficiency can result in significant physiological changes and specific illnesses that need medical attention.

While some hormonal abnormalities are persistent, others are transient (long-term). Additionally, certain hormone imbalances must be treated for you to maintain your physical health, while others may not have a direct influence on your health but still have a detrimental impact on your quality of life.

WHAT CONDITIONS ARE CAUSED BY HORMONAL IMBALANCES?

Hormone issues are the root of many illnesses. Most hormones have symptoms and health implications when there is too much or too little of them. While many of these imbalances need to be treated, others of them may just be short-lived and disappear on their own. The following are a few of the most prevalent hormone-related conditions:

Irregular menstruation (periods):

The menstrual cycle involves several hormones. As a result, irregular periods may result from an imbalance in any one or more of those hormones. PCOS and amenorrhea are two particular hormone-related diseases that lead to irregular periods.

Infertility:

For those whose gender at birth is determined to be female, hormonal imbalances are the main cause of infertility. Infertility can be brought on by hormone-related diseases such as PCOS and anovulation. Aside from physiological problems that influence fertility, such as low testosterone levels, people who are born men might also face these issues (hypogonadism).

Acne:

The main contributor to acne is blocked pores. Although there are various causes of acne, hormone levels, particularly throughout puberty, are a major contributor. When hormones become active throughout puberty, oil glands, particularly those in the skin of your face, are stimulated.

Hormonal acne (adult acne):

When hormonal changes cause your skin to generate more oil, hormonal acne (adult acne) results. This is especially typical for those who are in menopause, pregnant, or undergoing testosterone treatment.

Diabetes:

Diabetes is the most prevalent endocrine (hormone-related) disease in the US. In diabetes, your pancreas either fails to produce any or enough insulin, or your body fails to utilize it efficiently. Diabetes comes in a variety of forms. Type 2 diabetes,

Type 1 diabetes, and gestational diabetes are the most prevalent types. Diabetes has to be treated.

Thyroid disease:

Hypothyroidism (low thyroid hormone levels) and hyperthyroidism are the two primary kinds of thyroid illness (high thyroid hormone levels). Each ailment may have several different causes. Treatment for thyroid disease is necessary.

Obesity:

An imbalance of some hormones can cause weight gain in the form of fat accumulation because several hormones can influence how your body utilizes energy and sends signals that you need food. As an example, high levels of the hormone cortisol and low thyroid hormone levels (hypothyroidism) can both lead to obesity.

Signs and symptoms of a hormonal imbalance

Your general health is greatly influenced by your hormones. Consequently, a wide variety of indications and symptoms may point to a hormonal imbalance. Depending on whether hormones or glands are not functioning properly, your indications or symptoms may vary.

Any of the following signs or symptoms might be caused by common hormonal conditions affecting people of all genders:

- Weight gain
- A hump of fat between the shoulders

- Unexplained and sometimes sudden weight loss

- Fatigue

- Muscle weakness

- Muscle aches, tenderness, and stiffness

- Pain, stiffness, or swelling in your joints

- Increased or decreased heart rate

- Sweating

- Increased sensitivity to cold or heat

- Constipation or more frequent bowel movements

- Frequent urination

- Increased thirst

- Increased hunger

- Decreased sex drive

- Depression

- Nervousness, anxiety, or irritability

- Blurred vision

- Infertility

- Thinning hair or fine, brittle hair

- Dry skin

- Puffy face

- Rounded face

- Purple or pink stretch marks

Remember that there is no known cause for these symptoms. It's not always a sign of hormone imbalance to have one or a few of them.

Some of these symptoms can also be indicative of other recurring illnesses. So it's a good idea to consult your doctor if you notice any significant changes in your physique or energy levels.

Indications of a sex hormone imbalance in those born with a gender preference.

The sex chemicals estrogen and progesterone, which are produced by the ovaries, can be out of balance in people who were assigned female at birth (AFAB). Additionally, they may have too much androgen and testosterone. In AFAB people, an imbalance in sex hormones might result in the following symptoms:

- Acne on your face, chest, and/or upper back.
- Hair loss.
- Heavy periods.
- Hirsutism (excess body hair).
- Hot flashes.
- Infertility.
- Irregular periods.
- Loss of interest in sex.
- Vaginal atrophy.
- Vaginal dryness.

Sex hormone imbalance symptoms for people assigned male at birth

The following symptoms may manifest in people who were given the gender "male" at birth (AMAB) because of an imbalance of the sex hormones testosterone and other sex hormones:

- Decrease or loss of body hair.

- Erectile dysfunction (ED).

- Gynecomastia (enlarged breast tissue).

- Infertility.

- Loss of interest in sex.

- Loss of muscle mass.

Can hormone imbalance cause weight gain?

Yes, some hormonal imbalances can lead to weight gain, such as:

- Hypothyroidism: This illness develops when your metabolism slows down due to low thyroid hormone levels. Weight gain may result from this.

- Cushing's syndrome: This is an uncommon disorder that develops when your body produces an excessive amount of the hormone cortisol. Your face (also known as your "moon face"), tummy, back of your neck (often known as your "buffalo hump"), and chest all experience significant weight gain as a result.

- Menopause: Many people who were born female acquire weight during menopause as a result of hormonal changes that reduce their metabolism. It's critical to keep in mind that this kind of "hormonal imbalance" is normal and to be expected in life.

Other variables also play a role in weight gain. Consult your healthcare provider if you've gained weight unexpectedly or are worried about your weight.

Can hormone imbalance cause anxiety?

Yes, certain hormonal imbalances can cause anxiety, including:

Hyperthyroidism: Your body produces too much thyroid hormone if you have hyperthyroidism. Thyroid hormone excess supply accelerates metabolism. Along with unusual anxiousness, restlessness, and irritability, this might result in anxiety.

Cushing's syndrome: Cushing's syndrome (high cortisol) can result in anxiety, as well as depression and irritability, even though it's not a common symptom.

Adult-onset growth hormone deficiency: Anxiety and/or depression are frequently reported by adults with growth hormone deficiency.

Other diseases and circumstances might also contribute to anxiety. If you're anxious, it's crucial to speak with your health practitioner.

WHAT CAUSES MENOPAUSE

The end of a woman's menstrual period is known as menopause. Any changes you go through soon before or after your period ends, signaling the end of your reproductive years, might be referred to by this term.

Naturally declining reproductive hormones.

Your ovaries begin producing fewer estrogen and progesterone, the chemicals that control menstruation, as you enter your late 30s. As a result, your fertility declines.

In your 40s, your monthly cycles may get heavier, shorter, or more frequently as you get older. Eventually, on average at age 51, your ovaries stop producing eggs, and you cease having periods.

Surgery that removes the ovaries (oophorectomy).

The hormones estrogen and progesterone, which are produced by your ovaries, control the menstrual cycle. Menopause sets in right away when ovaries are removed surgically. Your period's end and you're likely to suffer additional menopausal symptoms like hot flashes. Due to hormonal changes occurring suddenly rather than gradually over many years, signs and symptoms might be severe.

Hysterectomy surgery, which removes your uterus but leaves your ovaries in place, typically does not result in an abrupt menopause. Your ovaries continue to release eggs and generate estrogen and progesterone even if you no longer have periods.

Chemotherapy and radiation therapy.

These cancer treatments have the potential to cause menopause, resulting in symptoms like hot flashes either during or just after the course of therapy. Following chemotherapy, menstruation (and fertility) may not always stop, therefore birth control may still be preferred. Only when radiation is focused on the ovaries can radiation treatment have an impact on ovarian function. Menopause won't be impacted by radiation therapy given to the head and neck, breast tissue, or other areas of the body.

Primary ovarian insufficiency.

Only 1% of women reach menopause before the age of 40. (Premature menopause). Primary ovarian insufficiency, which can be brought on by autoimmune illness or hereditary causes, is a condition in which your ovaries are unable to generate the appropriate amounts of reproductive hormones, which can lead to premature menopause. But frequently, there is no known cause for early menopause. To save the brain, heart, and bones of these women, hormone treatment is often advised at least until the age of menopause naturally.

WHAT IS CORTISOL

Your adrenal glands create the glucocorticoid hormone cortisol, which is then released into the body.

Hormones are substances that communicate with your organs, skin, muscles, and other tissues through your blood to coordinate various bodily activities. These messages instruct your body on what to do and when.

A particular class of steroid hormone is glucocorticoids. They regulate the metabolism of your muscles, fat, liver, and bones while reducing inflammation in all of your body tissues. The sleep-wake cycle is also impacted by glucocorticoids.

Your two small, triangular-shaped adrenal glands, or suprarenal glands, are situated on top of each of your two kidneys. The endocrine system in your body contains them.

Every organ and tissue in your body is impacted by cortisol, an important hormone. It performs a variety of crucial tasks, such as:

- Controlling the stress reaction in your body.
- Assisting in regulating your body's metabolism, which is how it uses fats, proteins, and carbs.
- Minimizing inflammation
- Blood pressure control.
- Control of blood sugar.
- Assisting in regulating your sleep-wake cycle.

Your body constantly checks your cortisol levels to keep them constant (homeostasis). Your health can be harmed by either higher or lower-than-normal cortisol levels.

Is cortisol a stress hormone?

Many people refer to cortisol as the "stress hormone." In addition to managing your body's stress response, it also has several other significant effects and functions throughout your body.

Additionally, it's crucial to keep in mind that, medically speaking, there are several types of stress, including:

- Acute stress: You experience acute stress when you are suddenly and briefly in danger. Examples of scenarios that result in acute stress include narrowly missing a vehicle accident or being pursued by an animal.
- Chronic stress: When you often encounter events that make you feel frustrated or anxious, this is known as chronic (long-term) stress. Chronic stress can be brought on by, among other things, having challenging or tedious work or a long-term sickness.
- Traumatic stress: When you encounter a situation that puts your life in danger and leaves you feeling terrified and powerless, you get traumatic stress. Traumatic stress can be brought on by, among other things, enduring a war, a sexual assault, or an extreme meteorological event like a tornado. These incidents may occasionally result in post-traumatic stress disorder (PTSD).

Your body releases cortisol when you experience any of these types of stress.

What does cortisol do to my body?

Your body's tissues all have glucocorticoid receptors. Cortisol can therefore have an impact on almost all organ systems inside your body, including:

- Nervous system.

- Immune system.

- Cardiovascular system.

- Respiratory system.

- Reproductive systems (female and male).

- Musculoskeletal system.

- Integumentary system (skin, hair, nails, glands, and nerves).

More specifically, cortisol affects your body in the following ways:

Regulating your body's stress response:

Your body can release cortisol in response to the release of "fight or flight" chemicals like adrenaline during stressful moments, keeping you on high alert. Additionally, during stressful times, cortisol causes your liver to produce glucose (sugar) for quick energy.

Controlling metabolism: Cortisol aids in regulating how your body uses carbohydrates, proteins, and fats for energy.

Suppressing inflammation:

Cortisol can temporarily improve your immunity by reducing inflammation. However, if your cortisol levels are regularly high, your body may become accustomed to having too much of it in your blood, which can cause inflammation and impair your immune system.

Regulating blood pressure:

Uncertainty surrounds the precise mechanism through which cortisol controls blood pressure in people. However, high cortisol levels can result in high blood pressure, and low cortisol levels can result in low blood pressure.

Raising and controlling blood sugar: Normally, cortisol balances the effects of the hormone insulin, which your pancreas produces to control your blood sugar. While insulin reduces blood sugar, cortisol elevates it by releasing glucose that has been stored in the body. Chronically elevated cortisol levels can result in ongoing high blood sugar (hyperglycemia). Type 2 diabetes may result from this.

Helping control your sleep-wake cycle:

In normal conditions, your cortisol levels are lowest at night before you go to sleep and are at their highest in the morning just before you wake up. This shows that cortisol is important for the start of wakefulness and affects the circadian rhythm of your body.

Having healthy cortisol levels is essential for survival and the maintenance of several body processes. Your general health may suffer if your cortisol levels are continuously too high or too low.

WHAT FOODS CAN LOWER YOUR CORTISOL LEVEL

Your body's release of cortisol typically peaks in the morning drops during the day and reaches its lowest level around midnight in your blood, urine, and saliva. If you work a night shift and sleep at various times during the day, this pattern may alter.

For most tests that measure cortisol levels in your blood, the normal ranges are:

6 a.m. to 8 a.m.: 10 to 20 micrograms per deciliter (mcg/dL).

Around 4 p.m.: 3 to 10 mcg/dL.

Normal ranges may differ from lab to lab, sometimes, and from person to person. Your healthcare practitioner will analyze the findings of the cortisol level test if you need one and let you know whether you require extra testing.

What causes high levels of cortisol?

Hypercortisolism, or prolonged experience of unusually high cortisol levels, is typically regarded as Cushing's syndrome, an uncommon illness. Cushing's syndrome and elevated cortisol levels can be brought on by:

The use of high doses of corticosteroid drugs, such as prednisone, prednisolone, or dexamethasone, to treat other ailments.

The adrenocorticotropic hormone-producing tumors (ACTH). Usually, your pituitary gland contains them. Rarely, neuroendocrine tumors in other organs, such as the lungs, can elevate cortisol levels.

Hyperplasia, or tumors of the adrenal glands, resulting in an overabundance of cortisol production.

What are the symptoms of high cortisol levels?

Your cortisol levels will determine how severe your Cushing's syndrome symptoms are. The following are typical warning signs and symptoms of elevated cortisol levels:

- Gaining weight, especially around the face and tummy.
- Fatty deposits between your shoulder blades.
- Abdominal stretch marks that are wide and purple (belly).
- You have thighs and upper arms with weak muscles.
- High blood sugar levels frequently progress to Type 2 diabetes.
- Elevated blood pressure (hypertension).
- Excessive hair growth (hirsutism) among those born with a gender preference.
- Fractures and weak bones (osteoporosis).

What causes low levels of cortisol?

Adrenal insufficiency is characterized by hypocortisolism or lower-than-normal cortisol levels. Adrenal insufficiency comes in two flavors: primary and secondary. Adrenal insufficiency can be brought on by:

- Primary adrenal insufficiency: The most frequent cause of primary adrenal insufficiency is an autoimmune response, in which your immune system unjustifiably attacks healthy cells in your adrenal glands. It is referred to as Addison's disease. A blood loss to the tissues or infection can potentially harm your adrenal glands (adrenal hemorrhage). These circumstances all restrict the generation of cortisol.

- Secondary adrenal insufficiency: ACTH production may be hampered if you have hypopituitarism, an underactive pituitary gland, or a pituitary tumor. Because ACTH tells your adrenal glands to produce cortisol, low ACTH also means low cortisol production.

Additionally, if you quit using corticosteroid drugs abruptly after a prolonged time of usage, you may experience lower-than-normal cortisol levels.

What are the symptoms of low cortisol levels?

Symptoms of lower-than-normal cortisol levels, or adrenal insufficiency, include:

- Fatigue.
- Unintentional weight loss.
- Poor appetite.
- Low blood pressure (hypotension).

Foods to Lower Cortisol

The value of a healthy diet cannot be overstated. The correct nutrients, especially those that reduce cortisol, can help manage a variety of health conditions. In general, it's a good idea to stay away from sugar, processed foods, trans fats, and sweetened beverages. These increase the number of oxidants in your body and add to your adrenal load, which can lead to inflammation, weight gain, mental health problems, and other problems.

Types of Foods to Lower Cortisol

It will be useful to understand how a few food types impact cortisol generally before looking at specific foods.

Carbohydrates

Many people will advise you to avoid carbohydrates, and frequently for good reason. But you should be cautious of processed carbs. On the other hand, complex, fiber-rich unrefined carbohydrates like whole grains and those in fruits and vegetables are healthy for you. Additionally, they contain the amino acid tryptophan, which is necessary for the brain to produce the sleep-inducing hormone melatonin. To have a decent night's sleep, you need this hormone. To repair itself, your body needs a sufficient amount of the correct kind of sleep. Therefore, don't be frightened to eat some whole grains.

Magnesium

Nearly half of all Americans do not get enough magnesium daily. Additionally, magnesium tends to be lost more quickly through perspiration and urine when you're under stress. Your stress levels rise when your magnesium levels are low. It can create a vicious loop.

By consuming meals high in magnesium, you can alleviate this problem. Great sources include avocados, some whole grains, and leafy green veggies.

Omega-3 Fatty Acids

Foods high in omega-3 fatty acids are among the foods that reduce cortisol. Low amounts of these fatty acids are often associated with greater cortisol levels in individuals. However, after they increase their omega-3 intake, they frequently see a decrease in the levels of this stress hormone. Foods high in omega-3s include flaxseeds, walnuts, and fatty fish like mackerel and salmon.

Probiotics

When coping with stress, maintaining good gut health is essential due to its substantial impact on overall health, immunity, and the gut-brain nexus. In summary, you need to take care of your gut flora since an imbalance might lead to health issues, such as an increase in cortisol. So foods strong in probiotics are foods to reduce cortisol. Sauerkraut, yogurt, kefir, and kimchi are some good examples.

The Best Foods to Lower Cortisol

These are the best foods to lower cortisol to add to your grocery list.

Dried Apricots

Dried apricots, which are high in magnesium, aid in muscular relaxation and reduce heart palpitations. Due to their rich vitamin C content, they help strengthen your immune system. Their abundant fiber promotes digestive wellness.

Fatty Fish

Omega-3 fatty acids found in fatty fish like salmon, mackerel, herring, cod, and sardines aid to regulate your cortisol and adrenaline levels. They support heart health as well.

Leafy Green Vegetables

The nutrients vitamin C, magnesium, and folate are found in leafy green vegetables including kale, spinach, cauliflower, and broccoli. Magnesium helps maintain cortisol levels, vitamin C is an excellent antioxidant, and Folate contributes to the brain's creation of dopamine and serotonin. Additionally high in vitamin K are collard greens. This vitamin is essential for maintaining healthy blood calcium levels, blood clotting, and bone growth. Significant levels of digestive-aiding enzymes may be found in microgreens and sprouts.

Whole Grains

It takes some time to digest whole grains. By doing this, they guarantee a regular, continuous release of serotonin, the hormone associated with happiness. Additionally, they support the stabilization of your blood sugar levels. Brown rice, quinoa, buckwheat, barley, oatmeal, whole-wheat bread, pasta, and crackers are examples of whole grains. Amaranth is an "ancient grain," much like quinoa. It has a lot of protein, fiber, and B vitamins.

Tea

Black or green teas are excellent substitutes for coffee and a rich source of vitamin C. According to research, black tea decreases cortisol levels. Green tea is also adaptogenic despite having a somewhat high caffeine content. This implies that it enhances your body's capacity to cope with stress and aids in the recovery of its physiological processes. However, if you're sensitive to caffeine and overstimulated, avoid drinking green or black tea since it may keep you up at night and put further stress on your adrenal glands.

Herbal teas with calming effects and sleep aids include chamomile, valerian, peppermint, and rose. Additionally, lemon balm tea may promote and enhance sleep while calming your sympathetic nervous system.

Eggs

Omega-3 fatty acids, choline, which supports brain function, and tryptophan, which promotes serotonin production, are all found in eggs.

Turkey

Tyrosine is also included in turkey, a rich source of lean protein. This amino acid aids in improving brain dopamine and norepinephrine levels, which improves focus.

Seeds and Nuts

Magnesium is found in abundance in seeds, which aid in emotional control. Flaxseed, pumpkin seeds, and sunflower seeds are easily available and simple to include in your diet.

Omega-3 fatty acids, which are found in nuts like walnuts and almonds, aid to decrease inflammation, support heart and brain function and lessen stress.

Fermented Foods

Probiotic-rich fermented foods like kimchi and sauerkraut benefit the gut flora and may lessen anxiety and sadness. Additionally, they include a variety of vitamins, such as vitamins A, B1, B2, and C. Additionally, foods that have undergone fermentation are high in antioxidants and amino acids.

Fruit

A lot of fruits are excellent diets to reduce cortisol.

The antioxidant lycopene helps stop the oxidation of cholesterol, while papaya, which is high in vitamin C, enhances the function of the adrenal glands. This indicates that it aids in preventing artery constriction.

Bromelain is an antioxidant and mineral found in pineapple. An enzyme for digestion with anti-inflammatory qualities is called bromelain. Vitamin C is also present in the fruit.

Avocados, a great source of healthy fats, also provide B vitamins, which support the health of the brain and nerves.

Antioxidants and anti-inflammatory cytokines may be found in large levels in blueberries and strawberries. These can aid in reducing the risk of stroke and heart disease.

Mangiferin is one of the several antioxidants found in mango. Super antioxidant mangiferin has potent antioxidative effects and may aid in the treatment of certain cancers.

Oranges, which contain a lot of vitamin C, might help you feel less stressed.

Magnesium, vitamin B6, and potassium levels in bananas are high. Potassium eases muscular tension and aids in the battle against depression. Additionally, this fruit possesses beta-adrenergic blocker characteristics. This indicates that it lowers your adrenaline levels. It is excellent for lowering stress levels because it contains tryptophan, which is necessary for the creation of serotonin.

Chocolate

Research suggests that dark chocolate may help lower cortisol levels. This delectable delicacy is low in caffeine and high in minerals including iron, copper, manganese, and zinc. Dark chocolate contains theobromine, which may give you a "feel-good" experience. Dark chocolate still includes a large quantity of sugar, therefore moderation is advised.

WHAT IS ESTROGEN

One of the two sex hormones that are frequently linked to cisgender women, transgender males, and non-binary persons with vaginal organs is estrogen. Estrogen, along with progesterone, is essential for the health of your reproductive system. Estrogen has a role in the development of secondary sex traits (such as breasts, hips, etc.), menstruation, pregnancy, and menopause.

Additionally, estrogen is crucial to various bodily processes. Because of this, while AFAB people produce the most estrogen, both genders do as well.

What are the types of estrogen?

There are three major forms of estrogen:

- The main type of estrogen that your body produces after menopause is estrogen (E1).
- During your reproductive years, the main form of estrogen in your body is estradiol (E2).
- It is the strongest estrogenic type. During pregnancy, the main type of estrogen is estriol (E3).

Where is estrogen located in the body?

During your reproductive years, your ovaries produce the majority of your estrogen. Adipose tissue (body fat) and your adrenal glands, which are located on your kidneys, both release estrogen. During pregnancy, the placenta, which is the organ that permits the exchange of nutrients between the mother and the fetus, secretes estrogen.

Once estrogen is released, it moves via your bloodstream to the area of your body that needs to be activated. There, estrogen interacts with an estrogen receptor protein to initiate the process. Your whole body has estrogen receptors.

What are the common conditions and disorders associated with estrogen?

The majority of illnesses that come under the category of women's health include estrogen. Among the most typical are:

- Anorexia nervosa: Low estrogen levels are linked to diseases like anorexia nervosa. Period irregularities and missed periods might result from low estrogen levels (amenorrhea). Little estrogen may also be seen in those who have very low body fat (such as models or athletes) or who have eating disorders.

- Breast cancer: Increased estrogen exposure does not raise the chance of developing breast cancer, according to studies, but it may make the disease worse after it has already started.

- Endometriosis: Endometriosis is not brought on by estrogen, although estrogen may make the pain from endometriosis worse.

- Female sexual dysfunction (FSD): Sexual pleasure may decrease as a result of physical and emotional changes brought on by declining estrogen levels. The use of estrogen for hormone replacement is not recommended until menopause.

- Fibrocystic breasts: During your menstrual cycle, fluctuating estrogen levels may cause your breast tissue to feel lumpy, sensitive, or painful.

- Infertility: Your menstrual cycle can be upset by both low and high estrogen levels. Infertility may be correlated with underlying factors that might result in low and high estrogen levels.

- Obesity: People with larger levels of body fat frequently have higher levels of estrogen.

- Osteoporosis: Your bones may become weaker due to low estrogen levels, making them more brittle and prone to breaking.

- Polycystic ovary syndrome (PCOS): When the ovaries create too many androgens, it results in PCOS (hormones associated with being assigned male at birth). Estrogen levels can occasionally be too high in PCOS when compared to progesterone levels.

- Primary ovarian insufficiency (also known as premature menopause): The ovaries in this syndrome abruptly stop generating eggs (before age 40). Your ovaries, therefore, fail to secrete the amount of estrogen that your body requires.

- Premenstrual syndrome (PMS) and premenstrual dysphoric disorder (PMDD): Unpleasant physical symptoms and mental swings might result from the menstrual cycle's periodic hormone fluctuations. PMS and PMDD may be brought on by drops in estrogen after ovulation.

- Turner Syndrome: Turner syndrome frequently has undeveloped ovaries, which causes low estrogen levels. As a result, those who have this illness could not have their periods or grow breasts.

- Uterine cancer (endometrial cancer): The lining of your uterus may thicken as a result of high estrogen levels. Cancer cells may eventually begin to multiply.

- Uterine fibroids and polyps: Fibroids and uterine polyps, which are benign tumors that develop when there is an excess of estrogen in your body, may be linked.

- Vaginal atrophy (atrophic vaginitis): Your vaginal lining may weaken and dry out if you don't get enough estrogen. Most women have vaginal shrinkage throughout menopause and post-menopause.

The influence of estrogen on ailments that affect other bodily systems is still being studied. For instance, gastrointestinal illnesses and several endocrine abnormalities have both been associated with estrogen.

What are normal estrogen levels?

Estrogen levels fluctuate during a lifetime. The variation is typical. For instance, it is typical for estrogen levels to increase during adolescence and decrease as menopause approaches. Estrogen levels often increase during ovulation so that your body can get ready for pregnancy. When the pregnancy alterations are unnecessary, it's typical for levels to drop throughout your period.

Consistently low or high levels might be an indication of an underlying problem that needs your doctor's attention.

WHAT ARE LEPTIN AND LEPTIN RESISTANCE

Adipose tissue (body fat) releases a hormone called leptin that aids in your body's long-term maintenance of a healthy weight. It accomplishes this by controlling appetite and causing satiety (feeling full).

Hormones are substances that communicate with your organs, muscles, and other tissues through your blood to coordinate various bodily operations. These messages instruct your body on what to do and when.

Leptin was discovered in 1994, but scientists are still researching it to fully understand all of its effects.

What is the function of leptin?

Your body uses leptin primarily to help maintain a stable balance between food intake and energy expenditure (expenditure). Leptin helps control energy balance and inhibit (avoid) hunger so that your body doesn't produce a hunger response when it doesn't require energy (calories).

Despite having leptin receptors in various parts of your body, leptin primarily regulates appetite and energy balance in your brainstem and hypothalamus.

Leptin works to change food intake and manage energy expenditure over a longer length of time to assist maintain your normal weight. It does not influence your hunger levels or food intake from meal to meal.

When you drop weight, leptin has a stronger impact. Your leptin levels fall when your body fat (adipose tissue) declines, which tells your body it's famished. This can cause more strong hunger and appetite, which can increase food intake.

Leptin is still being researched by scientists, who think it also has an impact on metabolism, endocrine system control, and immune system operation.

What is leptin resistance?

Your brain doesn't react to leptin as it should if you have leptin resistance. You don't experience fullness or satiety since leptin continually stimulates it. Even though your body already has considerable fat reserves, this makes you consume more.

Your body goes into starvation mode because leptin resistance seems to have low levels of leptin. Your brain lowers your energy levels and causes you to burn fewer calories while at rest to conserve energy.

As a result of increasing hunger and slowing metabolism, leptin resistance exacerbates obesity and leads to extra weight gain in the form of fat storage.

Currently, researchers are striving to create drugs that can combat leptin resistance.

What are the symptoms of leptin resistance?

Leptin capacity to reduce hunger or boost energy expenditure is reduced as a result of leptin resistance. Due to this, despite having enough or excessive levels of body fat, the major signs of leptin resistance are increased food consumption and a persistent sense of hunger.

Leptin resistance is only one of several conditions and variables that may cause these symptoms, though. Leptin is still being studied by scientists, who may subsequently find other signs of leptin resistance.

What happens when leptin levels are too low?

Having lower-than-normal leptin levels is quite uncommon (hyperleptinemia). Congenital leptin deficiency, a genetic disorder that inhibits your adipose tissue from producing leptin, is the major disease linked to low levels of leptin.

Without leptin, your body assumes it has no body fat, which leads to acute, irrational hunger and excessive food intake. Congenital leptin insufficiency thus causes class III obesity and delayed puberty in children. Additionally, it is linked to the following illnesses:

- Frequent bacterial infections.
- Hyperinsulinemia (excess insulin production).
- Fatty liver disease.
- Dyslipidemia (an imbalance of lipids, including cholesterol and triglycerides).
- Hypogonadotropic hypogonadism (low sex hormone levels).

How do I raise my leptin levels?

Unfortunately, since your leptin levels are inversely correlated with the amount of adipose tissue in your body, there isn't much you can do to increase them to reduce hunger and appetite.

According to one research, those who lack sleep had higher levels of the hunger-signaling hormone ghrelin and lower levels of the fat-burning hormone leptin. It's advantageous to your general health, in any event, to get the recommended amount and quality of sleep because it's crucial for many reasons.

Additionally, researchers are examining the connection between the hormone leptin and triglycerides, a kind of fat also referred to as lipids. High triglyceride levels appear to affect how leptin functions, according to some research, however, these findings are debatable. A diet intended to minimize triglycerides may help increase your leptin levels, according to some scientists, but not all of them.

METABOLISM AND BODY WEIGHT

The term "metabolism" describes the chemical reactions that take place in your body as it transforms food and liquids into energy. Energy is produced and released by a complex mechanism that mixes calories and oxygen. Body processes are fueled by this energy.

What does your metabolism do?

Even while your body is at rest, your metabolism continues to operate. It continuously supplies energy for essential bodily processes like:

- Breathing.
- Circulating blood.
- Digesting food.
- Growing and repairing cells.
- Managing hormone levels.
- Regulating body temperature.

Metabolism and weight

It could be tempting to attribute weight gain to your metabolism. Since metabolism is a natural process, however, your body has a variety of processes that control it to suit your particular demands.

Rarely, medical conditions such as Cushing's syndrome or having an underactive thyroid gland that inhibits metabolism might cause significant weight gain (hypothyroidism).

Unfortunately, gaining weight is a challenging task. Your lifestyle, including your sleep, physical activity, and stress levels, are probably influenced by a mix of your genetic make-up, hormonal regulation, diet composition, and surroundings.

The energy equation becomes imbalanced as a result of all of these causes. If you consume more calories than you expend or expend fewer calories than you consume, you will gain weight.

Everyone loses weight when they expend more calories than they consume, even though some people appear to be able to do it more rapidly and readily than others. By consuming fewer calories overall, boosting your calories burned through physical exercise, or doing both, you can lose weight.

WHAT CAUSES HUNGER PANGS

Hunger pangs, often known as pangs of hunger, are a normal response to an empty stomach. They make the stomach feel either empty or like it's chewing.

However, hunger pangs can occur even when the body does not need food. Other circumstances and settings that might cause hunger pangs include:

- Sleep deprivation
- Dehydration
- Eating the wrong foods

What are the causes?

There are many distinct causes of hunger pains or pangs in people. These reasons are listed here:

Hunger hormone

When the stomach is empty or when the next meal is approaching, the brain releases the hormone ghrelin.

To digest food, the body releases stomach acids when ghrelin is present. Hunger pains result from the stomach acids attacking the lining of the stomach if food is not eaten.

When given to adults, ghrelin has been proven to boost the desire to eat by as much as 30%.

Quality of food eaten

Even when the body doesn't require calories, hunger pangs might still occur.

This occurs as a result of ghrelin's interaction with the hormone that controls blood sugar, insulin. Falling insulin levels result in rising ghrelin levels, which in turn increase hunger.

Junk food has a high sugar and simple carbohydrate content. When consumed, it induces an increase in insulin levels and a rapid decline. Even if the food was just ingested an hour or two earlier, ghrelin then rises.

In this approach, consuming a lot of bad food might make you hungry and trigger a pang reaction in your body.

Dehydration

Because the feelings of hunger and thirst are so similar, many people are unable to distinguish between them.

Thirst can result in symptoms like:

- Stomach pains
- Shaking
- Irritability
- Lightheadedness

The environment

Some people have pains when they smell or see something. The aroma of freshly baked goods or cooking often causes bodily reactions in many people. On-screen or internet food images can also make your mouth wet.

Even while it may not be driven by a desire for food, this kind of hunger nonetheless results in very genuine bodily sensations, such as hunger pangs.

Lack of sleep

Sleep deprivation has long been linked to overeating and weight gain. It seems that a lack of sleep or sleep of low quality may be related to hunger pangs.

According to a 2016 study, sleep deprivation amplifies the effects of a hormone that makes consuming sweet, salty, and high-fat foods more enticing.

After consuming a meal that provided 90% of their daily caloric needs, the sleep-deprived study participants found it difficult to avoid junk food two hours later.

Emotional state

In rare situations, people may mistakenly interpret their brain signals for hunger as aches. When someone is experiencing a high level of emotion, this might happen.

According to research, stress and other unfavorable emotions might make it seem as though the body needs food right away, even if it doesn't.

Sometimes it might be easier to discern between emotional and physical hunger when your stomach is grumbling or growling. Only when the stomach is empty can the noises be heard.

Medication and medical conditions

In rare instances, medical disorders might contribute to hunger pains. For those who have diabetes, this is accurate since hunger increases when blood sugar levels drop.

If pains are present together with other symptoms, it may be an indication of an infection or digestive condition that needs medical treatment. Watch out for signs like:

- Diarrhea
- Dizziness
- Fever
- Headaches
- Nausea
- Vomiting
- Weakness

Some drugs, such as some antidepressants, may obstruct the release of ghrelin and hunger signals.

HOW DO YOU ELIMINATE HUNGER PANGS

Eat at regular intervals

Depending on when a person typically eats, ghrelin is released.

Following a timetable will guarantee that food enters the stomach in time to buffer the gastric acid that is secreted in response to ghrelin increases.

When out of the house, it might be useful to pack wholesome, low-calorie snacks like fruit and almonds in case it's not feasible to have a complete meal at a set mealtime.

Choose nutrient-dense foods

By deciding on nutritious meal selections rather than processed ones, you can prevent insulin drops.

Eat balanced meals that contain:

- Lean protein, such as beans, lentils, and skinless poultry
- Whole grains, including brown rice, oats, quinoa, and whole-wheat products
- Fruits and vegetables, including fresh, frozen, and canned (without added sugar)
- Healthful fats, are found in avocados, olives, nuts, and seeds
- Low-fat dairy products or dairy alternatives

Foods that are heavy in sugar, salt, saturated fats, and trans fats should be avoided whenever possible. White bread and white spaghetti are examples of refined carbohydrates that should be consumed in moderation or not at all.

Fill up on low-calorie foods

Some low-calorie foods are big in volume, which means they fill up the stomach but do not cause weight gain.

Ghrelin levels will decrease with satiety, reducing the sensation of hunger. Low-calorie, high-volume foods include:

- Salads
- Raw or lightly steamed green vegetables
- Homemade vegetable soups
- Green smoothies

Stay hydrated

Drink water all day long. Aim for 8 glasses every day. Avoid drinking excessive amounts of diuretic drinks like alcohol and caffeine, which cause dehydration.

Get enough sleep

It seems sensible to create a sleep schedule to prevent eating cravings brought on by lack of sleep. Aim to sleep for 7 to 9 hours each night by going to bed and waking up at the same time every day.

Practice mindful eating

Pay attention to the flavor and texture of each bite as you eat. Eat slowly and completely. Avoid watching television while eating.

Use distractions

If hunger pangs are not caused by a genuine desire for food, a person may strive to ignore them.

Distractions that work well include:

- Reading
- Dancing
- Exercise
- Working
- Socializing

A typical hungry response is a stomach ache. Although they may indicate a need for food, hunger pains can also be an indication of other conditions, such as dehydration, lack of sleep, and worry.

Since they often disappear when food is consumed, hunger pangs rarely need medical treatment.

Dieters may want to adopt measures to reduce their hunger pangs to reach their weight loss goals.

WHAT HAPPENS WHEN YOU IGNORE HUNGER PANGS

Do you know the difference between hunger and fullness? What is your reaction?

It's time to tune back in if you've developed the habit of ignoring your hunger cues or purposefully underrating when they appear.

If you've experienced times of constraint, you can't anticipate developing a bodyawareness instantly. It will take time for your perception to adjust since you have been rejecting your real, bodily sensations for a long.

Here's what happens when you get into the habit of ignoring your hunger cues:

1. You'll struggle to retain your energy since you won't be able to feel when you're hungry or full, making it more difficult to detect these indications.
2. You begin to want meals with little nutritious value. If you're disregarding your hunger, probably, you're not paying much attention to what food you might truly need to keep dancing.

It's acceptable to ignore early signs of hunger, such as low energy or a growling stomach, but you don't want to get to the point where you're so hungry that you feel dizzy or ill, can't focus, have a headache, or get irritable. Your body uses these early hunger cues to let you know when to eat, so learn to appreciate them. The secret is to eat every three to four hours and to only consume enough food to satisfy you without filling you up, leaving you feeling somewhat peckish right before your next meal or snack. Depending on how many meals (three) and snacks (0–3) you eat throughout the day, you should feel hungry three to six times a day if you're eating enough to feel satisfied and full.

If losing weight is your aim, eating three meals and two 150-calorie snacks per day may seem excessive, but nibbling between meals often results in less food being consumed at breakfast, lunch, and supper. The key to creating the calorie deficit you need to lose weight is to consume fewer calories overall each day since you aren't at all hungry during the day.

CAN DRINKING WATER HELP TO GET RID OF HUNGER PANGS

Did you know that persistent hunger feelings are one of the MAIN reasons so many individuals veer off track when dieting and trying to lose weight?

Even the strongest among us are vulnerable to them since their hunger may dominate our thoughts and sap our willpower almost to the point of nonexistence. When this occurs, we frequently grab the first thing we see, even though it's frequently not the healthiest option.

While sometimes "cheating" shouldn't be enough to convince you to give up your efforts to lose weight and get in shape, sadly, that's what so many people seem to do. A few slip-ups may easily lead to giving up and laziness.

Flush away fat and water weight

Drinking A LOT OF WATER is one of the most crucial things you can do to control hunger and permanently reduce those excess pounds. Drinking water throughout the day can help you remain on track so that you can achieve your objectives. Of course, eating frequent, wholesome meals is still necessary to keep your metabolism working at its peak.

The body may be cleansed of waste by consuming eight to ten 8-ounce glasses of water daily, and it can even act as an appetite suppressant. Additionally, it aids in the body's cessation of excessive water retention, which can aid in the loss of additional water weight.

Avoid falling into this trap

You may only be thirsty when you need to eat or drink anything. Reread that last phrase. So many people fall victim to the myth that they are HUNGRY when they are just thirsty.

Drink a glass of water first before grabbing something to eat, if possible. If you're still hungry after 15 minutes, you might want to get a healthy snack, but chances are good that your hunger will have subsided by then. One of the finest strategies you can use to battle those stubborn pounds is to carry a bottle of water with you all day and drink it when you start to feel hungry.

BENEFITS OF EATING HEALTHY

Maintaining a healthy weight, avoiding sickness, and improving your mood are just a few of the numerous health advantages of eating well.

In general, choosing real foods is the first step toward a healthy diet. Lean proteins, whole grains, healthy fats, and other nutrient-dense foods from all of the main food categories are included in a balanced diet, while processed foods should be avoided or drastically reduced.

Healthy Weight

The risk of many chronic health problems can be lowered by maintaining a healthy weight. However, being overweight or obese greatly raises your risk of developing major illnesses, such as:

- Heart disease
- Some cancers
- Type 2 diabetes
- Osteoporosis

Vegetables, fruits, and beans are just a few nutritious foods that are low in calories and high in beneficial elements. Additionally, they often include more dietary fiber. Dietary fiber is crucial for controlling weight. It aids in regulating hunger by prolonging the feeling of fullness and aids in elimination.

Other healthy eating advice for keeping a healthy weight includes:

- Plan your healthy meals to lessen your likelihood of errant decisions or binge eating.

- Be aware of how much you are eating because it is really simple to eat more calories than you think.

- Eat a variety of veggies to increase your feeling of satisfaction.

- Use herbs and spices; they enhance taste without adding a lot of calories.

- Check the nutrition information labels: Understand exactly what is in the meals you consume.

Better Mood

There could be a direct connection between nutrition and mood, according to research. Researchers discovered in 2016 that high glycemic load meals may exacerbate feelings of sadness and weariness.

Foods having a high glycemic load include simple sugars or refined carbs. Sugary beverages, white breads, biscuits, cookies, and cakes are a few examples of this sort of cuisine. Lean meats, whole grains, veggies, and whole fruit, on the other hand, have a reduced glycemic load.

Heart Health

The biggest cause of mortality for people in the US is heart disease, according to the US Center for Disease Control and Prevention. According to the American Heart

Association, approximately half of all adults in the country are affected by heart disease.

High blood pressure or early heart disease can be avoided with a healthy diet and more exercise. As a dietary strategy to lower high blood pressure, the Dietary Approaches to Stop Hypertension (DASH) diet is advised. This diet consists of:

- Eating lots of fruits, veggies, and whole grains.
- Take fish, poultry, legumes, nuts, and vegetable oils that are fat-free or low-fat.
- Reducing consumption of saturated and trans fats, which are found in foods like fatty meats and whole milk.
- Limiting consumption of foods and beverages with added sugar.
- Limiting your daily salt consumption to no more than 2,300 milligrams and boosting your calcium, potassium, and magnesium intake. Be aware that the optimal daily salt intake is 1,500 mg.
- Additionally, eating fiber-rich diets is advised for heart health. Dietary fiber may lower the risk of heart disease and other chronic illnesses and lower blood cholesterol levels.

Reduced Risk for Cancer

Antioxidant-rich meals can lower your chance of contracting some malignancies. To prevent disease-causing free radicals from harming our body cells, antioxidants must be present.

Numerous phytochemicals found in fruits, vegetables, nuts, and legumes serve as antioxidants.

Antioxidant-rich foods include:

- Seeds and nuts
- Dark leafy greens
- Berries, such as raspberries and blueberries
- Carrots and pumpkins

Improved Gut Health

Enough naturally occurring bacteria are present in a healthy gut or colon, helping with digestion, metabolism, and overall well-being. The gut microbiota is altered by an unhealthy diet that is heavy in sugar and low in fiber, which leads to more inflammation and poor health.

Prebiotics and probiotics, which support the growth of good bacteria in your gut, are provided by a diet high in fruits, vegetables, whole grains, and legumes and low in sugar.

Examples of foods high in pre/ probiotics include:

Fiber (a prebiotic)

Fermented foods rich in probiotics:

- Kefir
- Miso

- Yogurt

- Sauerkraut

- Kimchi

Improved Memory

According to research, eating well may help prevent cognitive impairment. Vitamin D, C, E, omega-3 fatty acids, fish, polyphenols, and flavonoids were all deemed advantageous in one research. The previously suggested healthy dietary practices in this article also aid memory.

Numerous healthy diets share the following characteristics:

- Consume extra veggies by packing half of your plate with them. Make sure to use a range of hues, and use enough greens.

- Consume fruit to get your fiber fix while avoiding juice.

- Consume whole grains; choose a range of high-fiber foods.

- Nuts and seeds are welcome.

- The best choices for fats include olive oil, olives, nuts, nut butter, seeds, and avocados.

- Consume lean protein: If you consume meat, make it lean and consume it in moderation. Include plenty of beans in your plant-based diet.

HOW TO BUILD SOME HEALTHY EATING HABITS

Many of us have ingrained patterns in our diet. Some are healthy (I always eat fruit for dessert) and some are not so healthy (I always treat myself to a sweet drink after work). It's never too late to change your eating habits, even if you've been following the same one for a while.

It should come as no surprise that your regular diet has a significant impact on your general health. You can be more productive at work and in life in general when you have a healthy body and mind. An essential component of living a healthy lifestyle is having a good diet. Your diet, when combined with exercise, can help you achieve and maintain a healthy weight, lower your chance of developing chronic diseases, and improve your general health. The following advice will assist you in beginning a healthy eating diet and lifestyle if you wish to start on this great path.

1. Balance your meals

Make sure to portion your food to prevent overeating.

To receive enough nutrients each day, your diet should be composed of 45 percent carbs, 30 percent protein, and 35 percent healthy fats.

2. Stay away from junk food

If you want to maximize your calorie intake, stick to eating whole, unprocessed meals.

The numerous artificial preservatives included in processed meals will make you feel sluggish all day.

3. Colorful food is good

Add lots of colorful fruits and leafy greens.

They are nutrient- and antioxidant-rich, which will increase your energy and motivate you to face the day.

4. Eat regularly

You'll overeat if you wait too long to eat.

To increase your metabolism and energy, strive to consume at least six modest meals (including healthy snacks) each day.

It's not as difficult to establish a healthy eating routine as you would believe. Although it requires a lot of self-control, it is possible and worthwhile. Anyone who recognizes the significance of eating a healthy diet will be inspired to choose their food wisely. You'll have the motivation and inspiration to take on any deadlines and responsibilities that come your way.

Short-term weight loss might result from drastic, rapid changes, such as eating nothing but cabbage soup. However, making such drastic adjustments is neither wise nor healthy, and it won't work in the long run. To change your eating habits for the better, use a deliberate strategy that includes reflection, replacement, and reinforcement.

- REFLECT on all of your specific eating habits, both bad and good; and, your common triggers for unhealthy eating.

- REPLACE your unhealthy eating habits with healthier ones.
- REINFORCE your new, healthier eating habits.

HEALTHY FOODS TO INCORPORATE INTO A DAILY DIET

One may increase their intake of vital nutrients by following a balanced diet that features foods from all the food categories.

Many people follow the same weekly menus and repetitive diets. However, including the following items in weekly meal plans can support their health and enable them to function at their peak.

One may, for instance, try a 2-week rotating meal plan and switch up their protein, veggies, and berries. This increases variation and nutritional diversity.

In this section, we'll look at some of the best meals to eat regularly. It examines what the science has to say about their health advantages and provides advice on how to eat them.

Lean protein

For healthy growth and development as well as to retain muscular mass, people require protein.

Each meal should contain protein to maintain blood sugar balance and prevent spikes that may result from eating only carbs. People's energy and focus may be maintained with the use of this strategy.

A person's protein requirements vary depending on their sex, age, and weight. In addition, a person's need for protein differs depending on how much and what kind of exercise they engage in as well as if they are pregnant or nursing.

According to the United States Department of Agriculture (USDA), the majority of Americans consume adequate protein, but they should choose leaner meat and poultry, increase their intake of protein-rich foods, and choose meat less frequently.

Adults require 5-7 ounces (oz) of protein daily, according to the USDA. Examples of popular, healthy protein foods and their protein contents are as follows:

- 1 sandwich slice of turkey = 1 oz
- 1 small chicken breast = 3 oz
- 1 can of tuna, drained = 3–4 oz
- 1 salmon steak = 4–6 oz
- 1 egg = 1 oz
- 1 tablespoon of peanut butter = 1 oz
- 1 cup of lentil soup = 2 oz
- 1 soy or bean burger patty = 2 oz
- one-quarter of a cup of tofu = 2 oz

To obtain a wide variety of amino acids and other crucial nutrients, people should aim to change their protein sources.

Broccoli and other cruciferous vegetables

Glucosinolates, which are sulfurous substances, are present in cruciferous vegetables. These are advantageous to your health.

One review from 2020 claims that glucosinolates control gene and cell pathways and may have anti-inflammatory and anticancer properties.

The substances could help treat and prevent metabolic syndrome, although additional study is required to confirm this.

The list of cruciferous vegetables that people should try to eat daily is as follows:

- Broccoli
- Cabbage
- Radish
- Cauliflower
- Broccoli sprouts
- Brussels sprouts

Cruciferous vegetables are a great source of fiber, as well as many necessary vitamins and minerals, in addition to sulfur compounds.

Arugula and watercress are two examples of leafy greens that contain healthy sulfur compounds.

Different colored vegetables

The Mediterranean diet is one of the healthiest eating patterns, according to health professionals like the American Heart Association (AHA).

Vegetable-focused diets, such as plant-based diets and the Mediterranean diet, can help reduce the risk of chronic diseases including diabetes and cardiovascular disease.

Eating a variety of colorful veggies every day makes it easier to receive enough phytonutrients, which are advantageous plant compounds.

Depending on their sex, age, weight, and level of exercise, individuals should consume 2-4 cups of veggies daily, according to the USDA's MyPlate webpage.

The USDA also recommends that consumers eat a variety of colorful plant foods, such as beans, lentils, and leafy greens.

Berries

People can meet part of their daily nutrient goals by eating berries.

One research from 2021, for instance, said that consuming 100 grams of raspberries, blackberries, or blueberries might satisfy more than half of an individual's daily needs for manganese, vitamins including vitamin C, and folate, and phytochemicals.

Berries are a great source of bioactive substances such as flavonoids, phenolic acids, and anthocyanins. These substances function as antioxidants, which may help reduce the risk of some cancers and prevent cardiovascular disease.

Berry foods to consume daily include the following:

- Blueberries
- Blackberries
- Raspberries
- Strawberries
- Cranberries

Fresh or frozen berries are better than dried types, which only have 20% as many phytonutrients.

Nuts

According to research, eating nuts regularly may be good for your health.

For instance, a 2019 prospective study involving more than 16,217 adults with diabetes discovered that those who consumed at least five servings of nuts per week had a lower risk of coronary heart disease, cardiovascular disease, and mortality than those who consumed less than one serving of nuts per month.

In particular, tree nuts were better at avoiding chronic diseases than peanuts.

One 2022 proposed that the high-fat content of nuts may discourage some people from eating them.

Nuts, on the other hand, are nutrient-dense foods with no negative effects on body weight, according to scientists. They might aid in weight loss when they take the place of other less healthful items in the diet.

Some people have allergies that prevent them from eating nuts. Nuts that are basic, unflavored, and unsalted are a healthy alternative for people who can consume them. Calcium, magnesium, and zinc are among the vital nutrients that may be found in all nuts.

One of the best food sources of the mineral selenium is Brazil nuts, which contain 95.8 micrograms per nut (mcg). This exceeds the adult daily need of 55 mcg by a considerable amount.

Olive oil

A staple of the Mediterranean diet is olive oil. Polyphenols are abundant in olives. These serve as antioxidants and defend the body from oxidative harm.

According to a 2021 study, phenolic chemicals found in olive oil may have anti-inflammatory and anticancer effects in test tube experiments.

The authors of this study hypothesized that persons who use less olive oil would benefit from using more, even if further human studies are required.

Olive oil that is extra virgin and unfiltered has the highest concentrations of beneficial polyphenols. Although it is often more costly, high-quality olive oil can be saved for pouring over salads and vegetables. It may be more efficient to cook with regular olive oil.

Summary

People may stay healthy and avoid developing some chronic illnesses by including lean protein, veggies, and nuts in their diet daily.

Compounds like polyphenols and glucosinolates, which are especially healthy, are present in some plant foods including berries and cruciferous vegetables.

A person may assist guarantee that they obtain a wide variety of important nutrients by incorporating these foods into a weekly meal plan, possibly on a two-week rotating schedule. It can also be more gratifying and enticing, and it prevents having a repetitive diet.

UNDERSTANDING PORTION SIZES

Portion size refers to how much food you are given or consumed. Meal to meal might have different portion sizes. For instance, you might just have two cups of popcorn at home, but movie theaters might provide a full tub drenched in butter.

Proper portion control is crucial whether you're trying to lose weight or just keep it steady. You may estimate how many calories you are probably ingesting by using portion control. You are consuming what your body requires to flourish rather than needlessly overindulging.

TIPS FOR CONTROLLING PORTION SIZES

Here are some useful suggestions for limiting portion sizes, both at home and when dining out, whether you're attempting to lose weight or even simply maintain your weight.

Use a smaller plate

The use of smaller serve ware and plates is one of the finest strategies to manage portion sizes. Utilizing smaller plates will create the appearance that a smaller piece of food seems larger, deceiving your brain into thinking that you have consumed more food overall.

Use your hands as a serving guide

It might be a bother to weigh your meals on a scale several times a day, especially if you spend most of the day away from home. Using your hands to measure your meal is an excellent method.

A serving of protein = 1 palm (~3.4oz)

A serving of vegetables = 1 fist (~1 cup)

A serving of carbs = 1 cupped hand (~½-⅔ cup)

A serving of fats = 1 thumb (~1 tbsp)

Ask for half portions

Large meal quantities are a common practice in restaurants. Many Americans overeat because most restaurants pile two to three times the advised serving size onto each dish. Some restaurants provide both large and small portions of menu items. If none of these choices are available, request a to-go box with your meal and save half of it for the following day. Some restaurants may even do this for you!

Unwanted weight gain may start with large portion sizes.

To control portions, you can take a variety of useful actions. With these easy adjustments, portions have been effectively reduced without sacrificing taste or sensations of fullness.

For instance, you may lessen your risk of overeating by measuring your food, using smaller plates, drinking water before meals, and eating more slowly.

At the end of the day, portion control is a simple solution that raises your standard of living and might help you avoid bingeing.

BENEFITS OF DRINKING ENOUGH WATER

How much water per day should you consume? You are surely aware of the need of staying hydrated when the outside temperature is high. No matter what the temperature says, though, staying hydrated is a daily need. Unfortunately, a lot of people, especially elderly people, don't drink enough. Thirst is less apparent to older persons than it was to them when they were younger. And if they are taking a medication like a diuretic, which can lead to fluid loss, that might be an issue.

Benefits of drinking water

Every system in the body needs water to function correctly. Water serves a variety of vital functions, including the following, according to the Harvard Medical School Special Health Report 6-Week Plan for Healthy Eating:

- Carrying nutrients and oxygen to your cells
- Flushing bacteria from your bladder
- Aiding digestion
- Preventing constipation
- Normalizing blood pressure
- Cushioning joints
- Protecting organs and tissues
- Regulating body temperature
- Maintaining electrolyte (sodium) balance.

You're staying hydrated if you're providing your body with the fluids it needs to perform those functions.

You run the danger of dehydration if you don't consume enough water each day. Weakness, low blood pressure, light-headedness, confusion, and dark urine are all warning indications of dehydration.

How much water should you consume? The average person needs four to six glasses of water each day.

How much water should you drink a day?

The four to six-cup guideline is for persons who are typically healthy. If you have certain medical conditions, such as thyroid illness or kidney, liver, or heart issues, or if you're taking medications that cause you to retain water, such as non-steroidal anti-inflammatory drugs (NSAIDs), opiate pain relievers, and some antidepressants, you might consume too much water.

If you fall into such a category, how much water should you consume each day? There is no universal solution. Individual water consumption needs to be considered, so if you're unsure of how much is best for you, talk to your doctor.

However, even a healthy person's water requirements might change, especially if you're exercising or outdoors on a hot day and are sweating a lot. Consult your doctor if you have questions about how much water to consume at such times, but as a general guideline, healthy individuals should consume two to three cups of water every hour, or more if they are perspiring significantly.

Tips for Avoiding Dehydration

You can stay hydrated without just drinking water. All liquids that include water help you meet your daily requirements. It's also a fallacy that drinking alcohol or caffeinated beverages dehydrate you since they induce you to urinate. They do, however overall, the water from these drinks makes a net positive contribution to the total amount of fluid consumed during the day.

Of course, there are a variety of factors that make water the superior option. Keep in mind that drinking sugary beverages can cause weight gain and inflammation, which can raise your chance of contracting illnesses like diabetes.

Caffeine overuse might make you jittery or prevent you from falling asleep. Additionally, men and women should each only have one or two drinks per day of alcohol.

Drink water gradually throughout the day to prevent dehydration. Having a drink with each meal, as well as socializing or using a medication, is a simple approach to do this.

And remember that meals high in water, such as salads, fruit, and applesauce, may also provide you with fluids.

BENEFITS OF DRINKING BLACK OR GREEN TEA

People throughout the world like drinking tea.

Camellia sinensis plant leaves are used to make both green and black tea.

The main distinction between the two is that black tea has undergone oxidation whereas green tea has not.

The oxidation process is sparked by rolling the leaves, which is the initial step in making black tea. The leaves turn dark brown as a result of this process, which also enhances and intensifies the tastes.

Green tea, on the other hand, is treated to stop oxidation and is thus considerably lighter in color than black tea.

To establish which type of tea is healthier, this section compares the studies on green and black tea.

Green tea contains high levels of the potent antioxidant EGCG.

Epigallocatechin-3-gallate, a powerful antioxidant, is abundant in green tea (EGCG).

Although green tea also includes other polyphenols like gallic acid and catechin, EGCG is thought to be the most potent and is most likely the source of many of green tea's health advantages.

The following is a list of potential advantages of EGCG found in green tea:

- Cancer. According to research conducted in test tubes, green tea's EGCG can kill cancer cells by preventing them from proliferating.
- Alzheimer's condition. The damaging effects of amyloid plaques, which build up in Alzheimer's sufferers, may be lessened by EGCG.

- Anti-fatigue. According to research, mice who drank drinks containing EGCG had longer swimming distances before becoming exhausted than mice that drank water.

- Liver defense. In mice fed a high-fat diet, EGCG has been found to prevent the formation of fatty liver.

- Anti-microbial. This antioxidant may even limit the spread of certain viruses and harm bacterial cell walls.

- Calming. Your body may experience a soothing effect as a result of how it interacts with receptors in your brain.

- The results provide credibility to the long-reported health advantages of drinking green tea, even though the majority of the research on the EGCG in green tea has been conducted in test-tube or animal experiments.

Black Tea Contains Beneficial Theaflavins

A class of polyphenols called theaflavins is specific to black tea.

They make about 3-6% of all the polyphenols in black tea and are created during the oxidation process.

Theaflavins appear to provide a variety of health advantages, many connected to their capacity as antioxidants.

These polyphenols may help your body's natural antioxidant production as well as shield fat cells from harm by free radicals.

Additionally, they could safeguard your blood vessels and heart.

Theaflavins have been shown in one animal research to lessen the risk of blood vessel plaque development by lowering inflammation and boosting the availability of nitric oxide, which causes your blood vessels to widen.

Theaflavins have also been demonstrated to drastically lower blood sugar and cholesterol levels.

They have been suggested as potential assistance in the control of obesity and may potentially increase fat breakdown.

Theaflavins in black tea may be just as potent an antioxidant as green tea polyphenols.

Black tea is the only source of theaflavins. They may help reduce weight and enhance blood vessel function due to their antioxidant effects.

Which one should you drink?

Green and black tea offer similar benefits.

Although their polyphenol compositions are different, they could have the same positive effects on blood vessel function.

The majority of studies suggest that green tea has more potent antioxidant qualities than black tea, however one study discovered that both types of tea were equally beneficial.

Although both types of tea include caffeine, black tea often has more of it, so green tea is preferable for those who are sensitive to this stimulant. In addition, green tea has higher levels of L-theanine, a relaxing amino acid that helps counteract the effects of caffeine.

Black tea, on the other hand, can be a wonderful choice for you if you're searching for a caffeine boost that is not as intense as coffee.

Remember that tannins included in both black and green tea can bind to minerals and hinder their ability to be absorbed. Tea may thus be best enjoyed between meals.

Black tea is ideal if you want a strong caffeine buzz even though green tea may have a slightly higher antioxidant profile.

Black and green tea both provide health advantages, including those for the brain and heart.

Although green tea may have stronger antioxidants than black tea, the research does not recommend one tea over the other.

Both include the soothing amino acid L-theanine as well as the stimulant caffeine.

In essence, both are excellent dietary additions.

BENEFITS OF VITAMIN SUPPLEMENTS

It might be difficult to get enough of the nutrients your body needs with today's hectic and contemporary lifestyle. Generally speaking, the body needs a certain quantity of vitamins and minerals to function. Each vital vitamin has a recommended daily allowance (RDA) for every person. For instance, the body needs vitamin K for calcium absorption and vitamin D for blood coagulation. Some nutrients may also promote physiological processes like the collagen and structural integrity of the skin.

The fact that vitamins are only a complement to the food you consume rather than a replacement for a healthy diet or antibiotics or other medications is one of the things to keep in mind while taking vitamins. For instance, you should continue taking the required medicines and combine them with the appropriate supplement, such as Luminance RED, if you have genital herpes. This is because to properly control herpes, a healthy diet must be accompanied by frequent usage of the appropriate vitamins and supplements.

Below are some of the many benefits of taking vitamins supplements:

1. Promotes Healthy Aging

No matter how much you wish you could live forever youthful, aging affects everyone. Additionally, you will need to take better care of your physical health as you age. Unfortunately, the body's ability to absorb essential nutrients decreases with age, and certain drugs may even cause nutritional depletion.

Taking vitamins is a quick and simple strategy to maintain good health. Numerous vitamins can assist restore your nutritional levels as you age and start to encounter deficits.

2. Reduces Anxiety and Stress

Your daily multivitamins contain minerals and vitamins that can dramatically lower stress and anxiety levels. B vitamins are used by the body to transform food into energy. These vitamins help maintain normal nervous system function. Daily vitamin intake may help your body's supplies of these nutrients refill.

3. Boosts Your Cardiovascular Health

Magnesium, CoQ10, and some vitamins, including the B vitamins and C vitamins, all support a healthy cardiovascular system. Therefore, taking vitamins may aid in maintaining heart health if you're one of those who are concerned about cardiovascular health in general. Just remember to pair it with heart-healthy food consumption.

4. Covers Your Nutritional Bases

Everyone tries to eat healthfully, but it can be challenging to receive all the nutrients you need from food alone. You can be confident that you'll fulfill your daily needs for all the necessary minerals and vitamins once you start taking vitamins regularly.

5. Supports Your Immune System

Your immune system is more crucial than ever in the present climate, so it only makes sense to attempt to nourish it as much as you can.

Vitamin C, which is well-known for being a potent antioxidant, comes to mind when you consider the vitamins typically linked to boosting your immune system. Additionally, you may boost your immunity by taking vitamins D and E.

Vitamins are available at your neighborhood drugstore or vitamin store. But depending just on these vitamins is insufficient. You still need to consume enough fruits and vegetables with green leaves.

6. Keeps Body in Good Working Order

Keeping the body healthy and functioning properly is one of the main advantages of taking vitamins daily. Vitamins work hard to maintain the body working normally and support vital daily functions.

Every nutrient you obtain from vitamins is on a mission to offer advantages that will hasten the achievement of your well-being goals.

7. Improves Your Eyesight

It has been proven that taking certain vitamins can promote eye health. Selenium, vitamins E, C, and A, and selenium help enhance vision. Zeaxanthin, lutein, and vitamin supplements can also reduce the risk of macular degeneration.

One of the main causes of bad vision in the majority of people is the growing amount of time spent staring at displays on TVs, computers, and mobile devices. For instance, your eyes would most certainly suffer if you spend 8 hours a day in front of a computer.

Taking preventative measures and routinely taking vitamins are effective ways to fight eyesight deterioration. Eating the right foods for your eyesight or eye health is also a wise choice, especially if you don't take vitamins consistently or sometimes forget to do so.

8. Keeps Your Bones Strong

You undoubtedly already know how important calcium is for strong bones. But did you know that calcium needs vitamin D to function properly?

After being exposed to direct sunshine, the skin also manufactures vitamin D, although the use of sunscreen, poor skin absorption and weak winter sunlight may inhibit the creation of this crucial nutrient. Even though milk has vitamin D added, most individuals don't frequently consume dairy products.

9. Aids Brain Function

The possibility that vitamins will aid to enhance brain function is another advantage. As other disorders like sadness and anxiety may be caused by vitamin shortages, it may also promote greater mental health. It is thus not harmful to take vitamins that might assist make up for such shortages. Just be sure you only take high-quality vitamins. Ask your doctor for advice if you're unsure of which vitamins are ideal for you to take.

10. Supports Healthy Metabolism

Your body uses certain enzymes and B vitamins, including riboflavin, thiamin, B6, B12, biotin, and folate, to digest fats, carbs, and protein for energy. Maintaining a healthy metabolism is important for your general health and good aging, and it may be done by eating well and exercising often.

11. Promotes Healthier Skin and Hair

The development of better hair and skin is one advantage of taking vitamins. There are certain vitamins, often vitamins E, A, and C, that aid minimize such issues if you're having skin issues, such as eczema, dry skin, or acne.

The greatest vitamins to take to develop fuller hair are B3 and C if you have split ends or thinning hair.

Vitamin intake has several positive effects on health and general wellbeing. They can help you achieve your wellness and health objectives by completing the nutrients you obtain from meals. But only if you remember to take your vitamins regularly and mix them with a nutritious, well-balanced diet will you be able to enjoy the advantages mentioned above.

HOW TO MANAGE HEALTHY HEART HABITS

Your strongest line of defense against heart disease, as well as one that might help you avoid heart attack and stroke, is to adopt healthy habits. Some of the finest actions you can do to maintain a healthier heart include:

1. Manage your blood pressure

The heart must work constantly to adjust for high blood pressure. Discuss the strategies you may take to decrease your numbers with your doctor if your blood pressure is persistently greater than 130/80.

2. Control your cholesterol

Exercise and a balanced diet can lower cholesterol levels. Reduce your intake of processed and fried meals as one strategy for lowering cholesterol. Increase your intake of whole grains, plant-based meals, and foods low in saturated fat to replace them.

3. Lose weight

If you are overweight, even a 10% weight loss will decrease your cholesterol and blood pressure. It may also lower your chance of developing diabetes. To determine a goal weight, consult a cardiologist or your doctor.

4. Exercise

Ideally, you should work out five times a week for at least 30 minutes. But if you're short on time, even increasing your movement in 10-minute increments might be beneficial. Every inch matters. Take a quick stroll after supper, or dance while you're preparing meals or washing clothes.

5. Stop smoking

Smoking is one of the worst things you can do to your heart. Just one cigarette a day increases your chance of developing heart disease, as well as other chronic conditions.

6. Calm down

Stress is not good for you. It's likely that if you're stressed, your heart is, too. Stress has detrimental consequences on your body's health in addition to encouraging harmful behaviors like smoking, consuming alcohol, and overeating. When you're feeling stressed or overwhelmed, we are aware that it's not always simple to calm down. Sometimes life is hectic! However, one method of finding inner peace is via meditation.

Healthy behaviors are essential for maintaining your heart in excellent condition. These will support your heart's health, increase its efficiency, and shield it from developing heart disease.